Essential Oils

Amazing Lifelong Secrets for Weight Loss, Beauty and Health

Table of Contents

Introduction

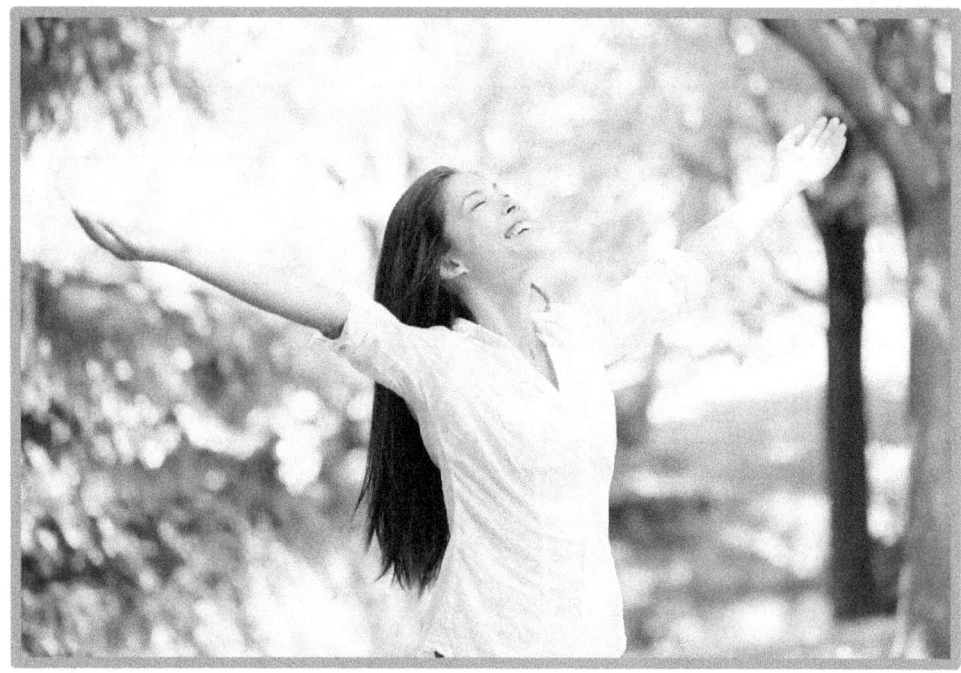

Whether or not you pay attention to the latest health and fitness trends, you have probably heard of essential oils. Essential oils come in little colored bottles that can be purchased from your local health food store or online from a supplier. While these oils do not have magical powers, they can provide some pretty significant benefits for your health and wellness. For example, lemon essential oil can be used as a natural cleaning product and it is known for its detoxification benefits. Lavender oil is commonly used in aromatherapy but can also help to improve the health of your skin.

If you are curious about essential oils, this is the right book for you. In this book you will learn all about what essential oils are and where they come from. You will read about the methods used to extract these oils as well as some unique uses for these oils that you may never have considered. Throughout the book you will receive recommendations for using certain oils to support healthy weight loss, to improve your skin and hair, and to treat minor ailments.

Here is a quick breakdown of what you will receive in this book:

- Overview of essential oils including production methods
- Explanation of common uses for essential oils

- Safe handling tips for essential oils
- In-depth explanation of 5 essential oils for weight loss
- Recipes for weight loss wraps and smoothies
- In-depth explanation of 5 essential oils for beauty
- Recipes for essential oil face wash and scrub
- In-depth explanation of essential oils for health
- List of other uses for essential oils including bug spray recipe

This is only a brief look at what you will receive in reading this book. If you are ready to learn about the benefits of essential oils, don't wait any longer. Get started!

Chapter One: What Are Essential Oils?

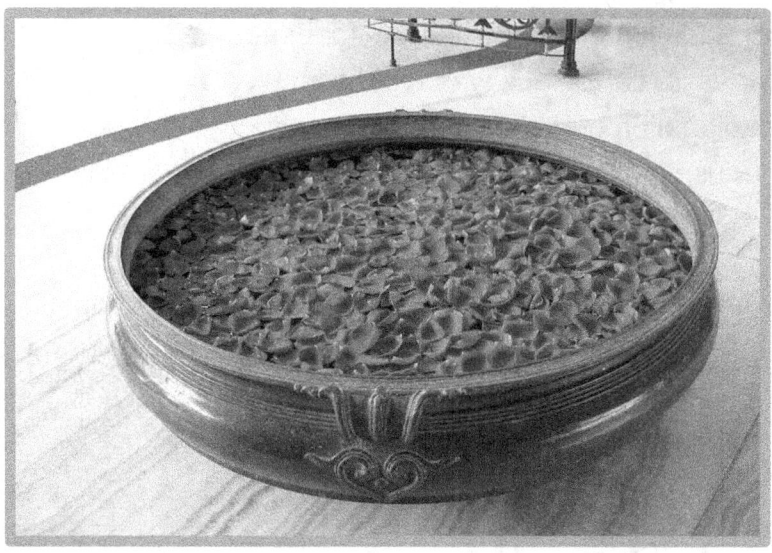

The term "essential oil" refers to the concentrated liquid that can be extracted from plants which contains volatile aroma compounds. In short, an essential oil is the "essence" of a plant because it carries the plant's scent. Other names for essential oil include volatile oil, ethereal oil and aetherolea but the term "essential oil" is used most commonly. Despite the name, essential oils are not true oils because they do not contain any fatty acids – rather, they are a hydrophobic liquid that can be extracted from plants through a variety of means.

Some common essential oils you are likely familiar with:

- Lavender oil
- Rose oil
- Eucalyptus oil
- Jasmine oil
- Cedar oil
- Lemon oil

Essential oils are wonderfully versatile, useful in a variety of ways beyond simply smelling good. If you are curious about the other uses for essential oils, keep reading!

Common Uses for Essential Oils

You are probably already a little familiar with essential oils in one of their most common forms – as an ingredient in spa treatments or bath and body products. As you already know, essential oils contain the aroma compounds of the plant so they are often used to scent beauty products. There is an entire industry devoted to aromatherapy which incorporates the use of essential oils primarily for their aroma, or scent. For thousands of years essential oils have been valued for their cosmetic properties, including their scent. What you may not realize is that their value goes way beyond their use in aromatherapy – essential oils also have benefits for weight loss, beauty and overall health.

Some other uses for essential oils include:

Restoring balance in the body – in many cases, our modern lifestyles leave much to be desired in terms of fostering physical wellness and balance in the body. Everything from poor diet to lack of exercise has an effect on the body, diminishing your energy stores and increasing your body's toxic load. Certain essential oils like tangerine, chamomile and spearmint can help to cleanse the body to restore balance.

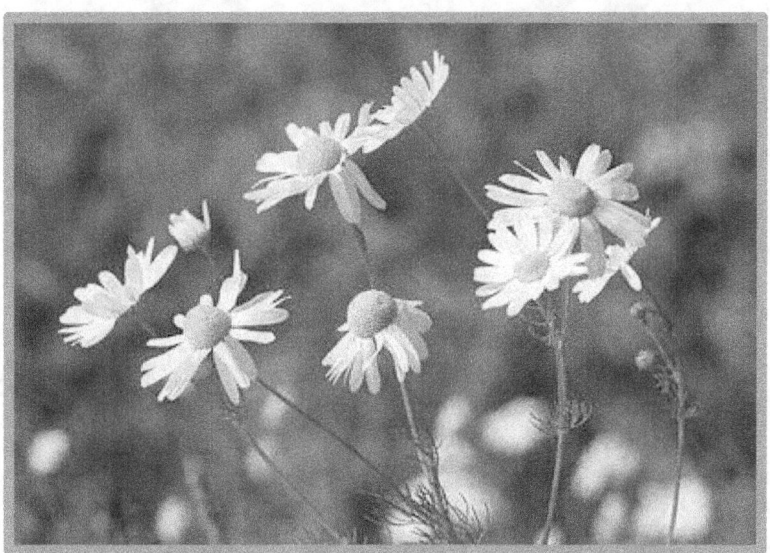

1: Chamomile

Promoting a positive emotional state – studies have shown that certain fragrances can active the limbic system (the part of the brain that is responsible for emotion and memory) which can affect your mood. Essential oils like lavender, citrus and peppermint have been shown to lift the spirits and to encourage a sense of wellbeing. The best way to use essential oils for this purpose is to use them in a bath or massage – you can also enjoy them through diffusion or inhalation.

All-natural cleaning products – you don't have to spend a lot of money on fancy cleaning products that are made with toxic chemicals just to keep your house clean. Several essential oils including lemon, thyme and lemongrass are great natural cleaning products that will leave your home smelling fresh. These oils have also been shown to repel insects and to polish countertops and other surfaces without leaving residue.

Improving skin health and clearing complexion – many modern beauty products are loaded with chemicals and artificial ingredients that can actually do more harm than good. Essential oils like vanilla, lavender and frankincense can help to clear your complexion and support healthy cell growth by all-natural means. These oils may also help to reduce the signs of aging and to promote healthy hair.

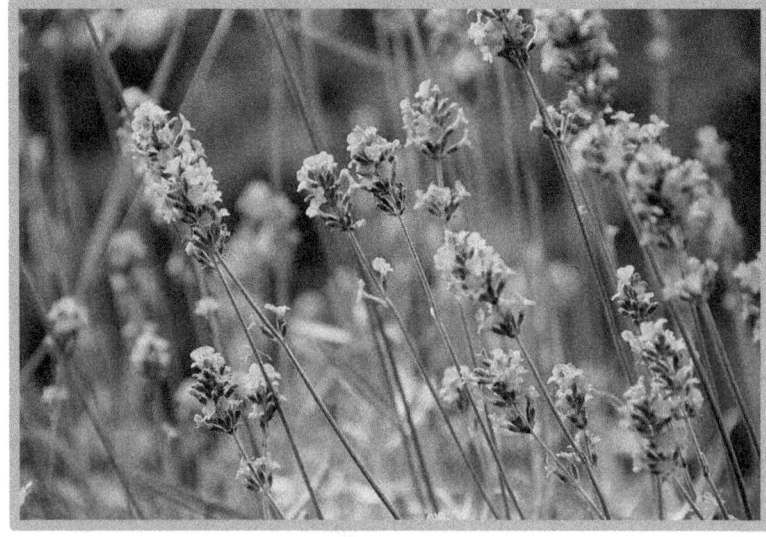

2: Lavender

Heightening spiritual awareness for meditation – for thousands of years, essential oils have been an important part of spiritual and religious ceremonies. In addition to helping you achieve a relaxed state of mind, certain oils like sandalwood, rosewood and hyssop may help you to transcend trivial thoughts and to achieve a spiritual state of mind. When used for this purpose, essential oils are typically applied directly to the body on the wrists, feet and behind the ears.

Ingredients in folk medicine remedies – folk medicine has been practiced for centuries to treat minor injuries and ailments including coughs and colds as well as bruises, sore throat and burns. Essential oils can be used to make tinctures and ointments for the treatment of minor ailments – baths treated with essential oils are also popular in folk medicine.

Essential Oil Production Methods

Now that you know the basics about essential oils including what they are and how they can be used, you may be curious to know where they come from and how they are produced. Essential oils can be extracted from the plant by a variety of methods including distillation, expression and solvent extraction. Below you will find a brief explanation of each of these extraction methods as well as a list of some of the oils that are most commonly produced using each method.

Distillation

The distillation process involves placing raw plant materials in a special distillation apparatus over water. This apparatus is commonly called an alembic and it is an alchemical still that consists of two separate vessels connected by a tube. The raw materials are placed in the main vessel which is then set over a container of boiling water. As the water boils, it heats the raw materials and causes them to release vapor. The vapor rises to the top of the alembic and cools upon making contact with the solid wall of the device. As the vapor cools and condenses it turns into a liquid which runs down the spout or tube into the second vessel for collection.

Commonly used for: lavender, peppermint, eucalyptus

Raw materials used: flowers, leaves, wood, bark, root, seeds

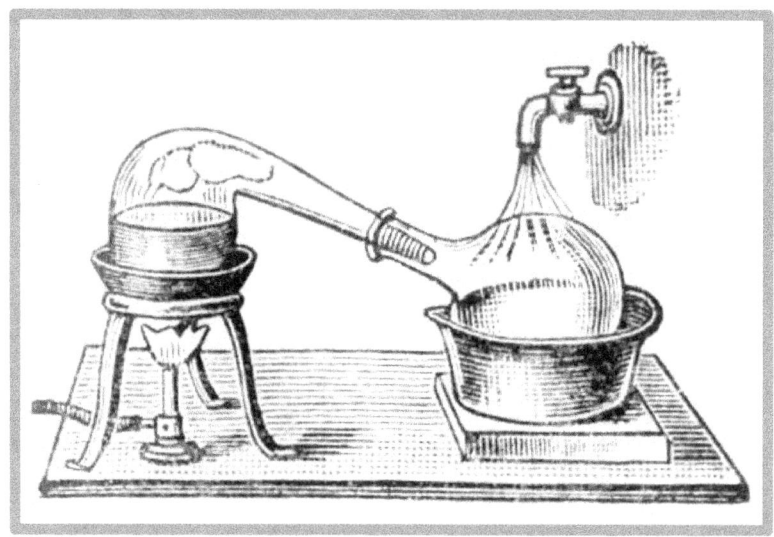

Expression

The process of expression involves physically pressing or squeezing the essential oil out of the raw materials. This extraction method is most commonly used for citrus like orange and lemon because the peel contains such a large quantity of oil. The two most common methods of expressing are mechanical or cold-pressing. Interestingly, though distillation is the most common form of essential oil extracting now, extracting used to be the only method available.

Commonly used for: citrus (lemon, orange, tangerine)

Raw materials used: peels, flowers, leaves, root

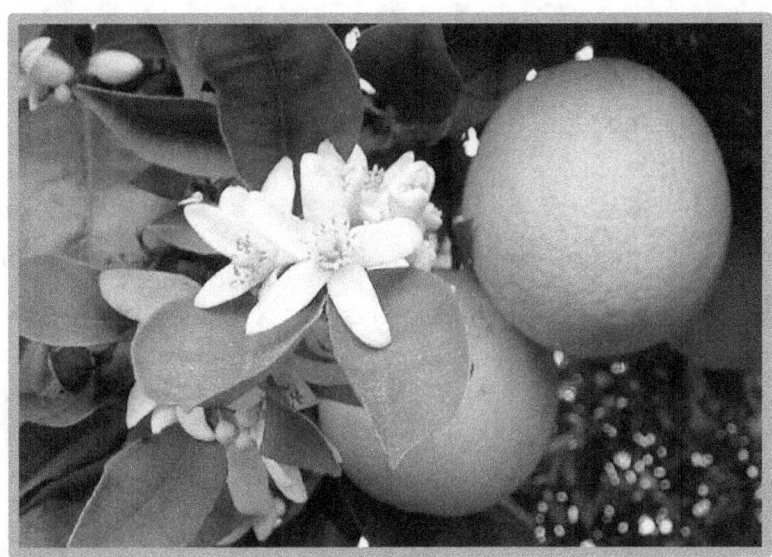

Solvent Extraction

In some cases (as with flowers), the raw materials are too delicate to extract by expression and the chemical components may be too easily denatured when exposed to heat during distillation. For these materials, the best extraction method is to use a solvent such as hexane or supercritical carbon dioxide, though ethyl alcohol is also commonly used. To extract the essential oil, a solvent is created using one of the two chemicals listed previously – this combination is called a 'concrete'. When alcohol is used to create a concrete, it can be removed by evaporation which leaves only the essential oil – in this case, called the 'absolute'.

Commonly used for: lavender, rose, hyssop

Chapter Two: Essential Oil Safety Tips

Essential oils are all-natural so you do not have to worry about whether they contain harmful toxins or chemicals like many commercial beauty products do. There are, however, some guidelines you should follow in using these oils. Below you will find some helpful tips to ensure your safety in using essential oils.

General Safety Tips

- Always read and follow instructions and warnings on essential oil labels

- Keep the oils out of reach of children and pets

- Do not apply any undiluted essential oils directly to the skin – they should be diluted with a carrier oil

- Always test the diluted oil on the skin of your inner arm to check for a reaction (such as redness or inflammation)

- Keep essential oils away from heat and flame (they are flammable)

- Do not ingest essential oils unless directed by a physician

- Keep essential oils out of your eyes, nose and mouth – essential oils are for external use only

- Do not use essential oils if you suffer from a heart or kidney condition until you check with your physician

Handling Spills and Accidents

Safe handling of essential oils is incredibly important – some of them are so potent that a spill must be handled as if it were hazardous. This is true of tea tree oil which, if spilled, should not be allowed to enter the sewer or a waterway. If essential oils are spilled, they should be absorbed with some kind of inert material and disposed of in a sealed container. If you get any essential oil in your eyes you should flush them immediately with cool water. Always wash your hands after handling essential oils and be sure to use soap to help dilute the oil.

Chapter Three: Essential Oils for Weight Loss

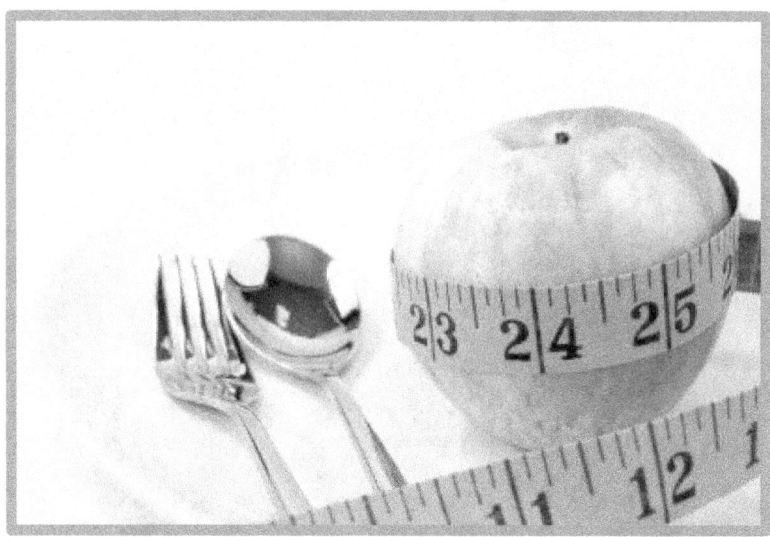

While no product can produce magical or instantaneous results, essential oils have been shown to support healthy weight loss. When it comes to losing weight, studies have shown that a holistic approach is best – you cannot expect to spot-reduce a certain part of your body or add/subtract something from your diet to cause the pounds to melt away. It took time and the combination of many factors to gain the extra weight you now carry, so you shouldn't expect to find some miracle cure to make it disappear overnight. Even if you could, research shows that slow weight loss is healthier and more sustainable in the long run.

When I comes to choosing essential oils to support your weight loss efforts, there are a few things to think about. First, you want to choose oils that will help to balance your appetite and to reduce cravings – if you snack less during the day your overall calorie count will be reduced. Second, look for something that boosts your metabolism to ensure that the food you do eat is being properly digested and absorbed by your body. Finally, essential oils for weight loss should increase your energy and lift your spirits so you have the energy you need to get your daily exercise.

Some essential oils recommended for weight loss include:

- Grapefruit
- Lemon
- Ginger
- Peppermint
- Cinnamon

Grapefruit

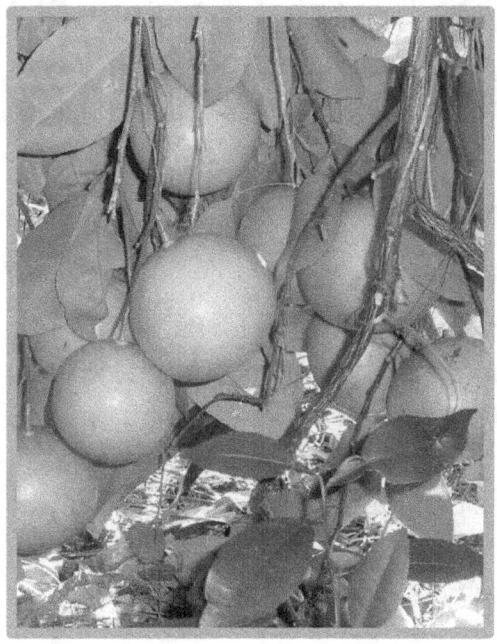

Grapefruit essential oil is extracted from the rind of grapefruits, the fruit of the Citrus paradise tree. The oil has a fresh, citrus aroma that has been shown to improve energy and to life the spirits – two things that are important while you are trying to lose weight. Other citrus oils in addition to grapefruit oil are also beneficial for weight loss.

In addition to promoting healthy weight loss, grapefruit essential oil is also very beneficial to the skin. The oil is very rich in d-limonene, a powerful antioxidant, which adds moisture to the skin, helping to firm and lift.

How to Use: To use grapefruit essential oil, it is recommended that you take 2 drops in a capsule up to three times per day. If you are using this oil for its skin benefits, dilute it in olive oil and rub it directly into the skin.

Components: Limonene, Alpha Pinene, Sabinene, Myrcene, Geraniol, Citronellal, Linalool, Decyl Acetate, Terpinenol and Neryl Acetate

Other Uses: In addition to its uses in supporting healthy weight loss, grapefruit essential oil also acts as a natural diuretic. When used as a diuretic, grapefruit essential oil can help to increase urine production, thus supporting the removal of toxins as well as excess water from the body.

Blend With: blends well with bergamot, frankincense, geranium and lavender

Lemon

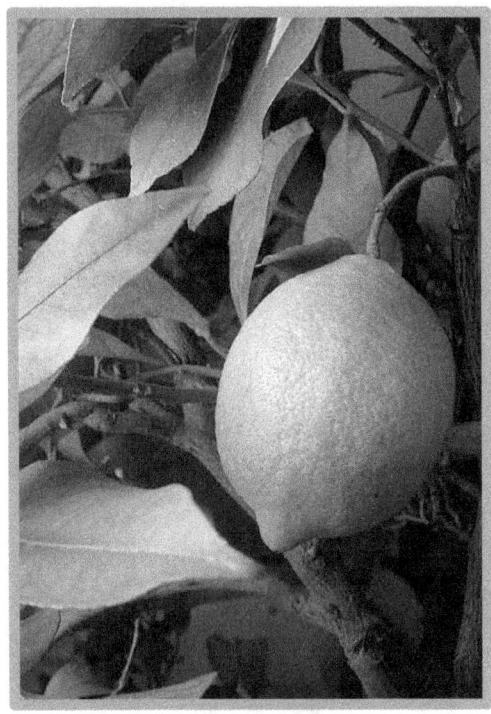

Lemon essential oil comes from the fruit of the lemon tree, *Citrus limon*. These trees are native to Asia and are known for their yellow color and sour taste. The essential oil is extracted by cold-pressing lemon peel.

Lemon, in all its forms, is known for its detoxification benefits. As you take toxins into your body through the food you eat, the air you breathe and the products you use, much of those toxins are stored in the body (primarily in fat). Detoxifying your body helps to flush those toxins which restores your body to its normal function.

How to Use: In regard to weight loss, lemon essential oil helps to flush stored toxins from the body, thus restoring your body to its normal function. To get the most benefit from this oil, ingest 1 drop per day in 4 ounces of liquid like water or tea.

Components: A-Pinene, Camphene, B-Pinene, Sabinen, Myrcene, Limonene, Nerol, Neral, Trans-a-Bergamotene, and A-Terpinene

Other Uses: In addition to its detoxification benefits, lemon is also known for relieving stress, anxiety and mental fatigue. This essential oil can help to promote a healthy and positive mindset which is very important while you are trying to lose weight.

Blend With: blends well with lavender, rose, sandalwood, geranium and tea tree oils

Ginger

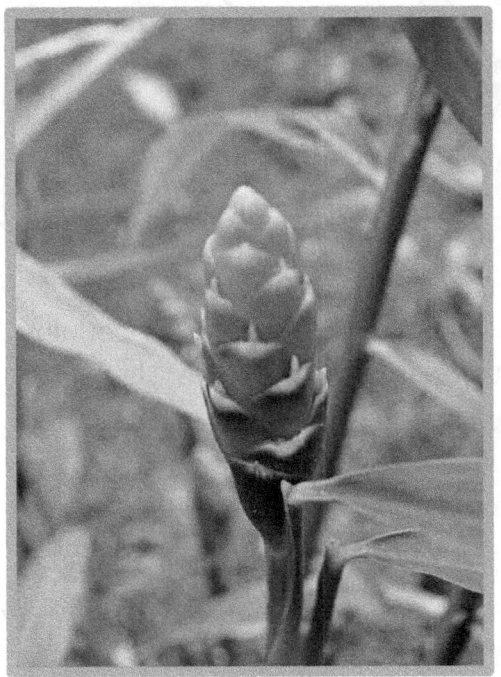

Also known as ginger root, ginger is the rhizome of the plant called *Zingiber officinale*. Though commonly used for culinary purposes, ginger also has a variety of medicinal benefits. This plant belongs to the same family as turmeric, cardamom and galangal.

Ginger essential oil is known primarily for its digestive benefits – it helps to stimulate the digestive system so that nutrients are properly digested and absorbed. It may also serve as a tonic to help promote detoxification.

How to Use: To use ginger as a weight loss supplement, it is best to ingest it. Dilute one drop of ginger essential oil in 4 ounces of liquid such as water, milk or tea.

Components: Gingerol, Sesquiterpenoids, Zingiberene, Bisabolene, Farnesene, Cineol, Citral and ß-phelladrene

Other Uses: In addition to supporting weight loss efforts by improving digestion, ginger essential oil can also be used to treat cardiac and respiratory disorders. Ginger is a natural expectorant which may help in treating colds, asthma and flu symptoms. In regard to its cardiac benefits, ginger helps reduce cholesterol levels and supports healthy blood flow.

Blend With: blends well with lemon, cedar, lime, eucalyptus, frankincense, geranium, rosemary, sandalwood, bergamot and orange

Peppermint

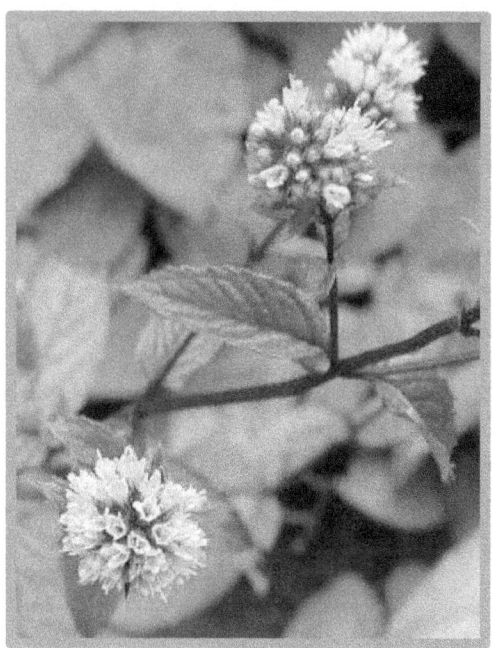

Peppermint essential oil is extracted from the peppermint plant (*Mentha piperita*) which is a hybrid of the watermint and spearmint plants. This herb is indigenous to Europe, though it is widely cultivated around the world.

In addition to its weight loss benefits, peppermint oil is very useful for skin and hair care. Use of peppermint oil in hair-care products can help to remove dandruff and lice while also soothing dry skin on the scalp. Peppermint oil may also nourish dry skin and reduce oil production.

How to Use: Peppermint oil provides weight loss benefits primarily by improving digestion – if your body does not properly digest and metabolize your food, you may end up storing more calories as fat. Peppermint oil can also help to improve your mood and increase your motivation. To use peppermint oil, dilute 1 drop in 4 ounces of liquid such as herbal tea. You can also rub several drops on the abdomen to help ease digestive discomfort.

Components: Menthol, Menthone, Menthyl Esters, Menthyl Acetate, Menthofuran, Cineol, Pulegone, Caryophyllene, Pinene and Limonene

Other Uses: In addition to its benefits for weight loss, peppermint oil has also been shown effective as a treatment for irritable bowel syndrome. A research study conducted in Italy revealed that patients who took peppermint oil capsules experienced a major reduction in symptoms compared to those who took the placebo.

Blend With: eucalyptus, rosemary, lemon and marjoram

Cinnamon

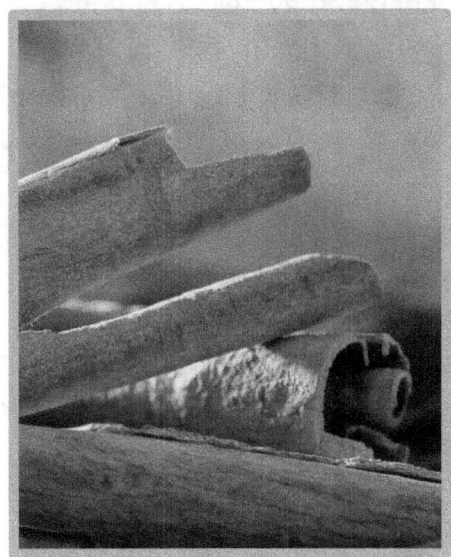

The spice known as cinnamon is derived from the inner bark of several trees within the genus *Cinnamomum*. The aroma for which this spice is known actually comes from the essential oil which can be extracted only by pounding the bark, macerating it in sea water and then distilling it.

The resulting oil is yellow in color with a very hot flavor and the characteristic cinnamon odor. As the oil ages, it may darken in color.

How to Use: Also referred to as Cinnamon Bark essential oil, cinnamon oil is primarily beneficial for weight loss in that it boosts the efficacy of the other recommended oils. This particular oil helps to detoxify the body while also improving digestion and blood circulation. To use this oil, dilute one drop in 4 ounces of water once a day.

Components: Camphor, Eugenol, Cinnamyl Acetate, Cinnamaldehyde, Beta-Caryophyllene, Linalool, Methyl Chavicol and Ethyl Cinnamate

Other Uses: In addition to its benefits for weight loss, cinnamon also provides a number of medicinal benefits. This oil is useful in treating respiratory orders and for promoting cardiac health. It has often been used to relieve menstrual discomfort and to ease digestive stress.

Blend With: blends well with lemon, rosemary, geranium, lavender and cardamom

General Weight Loss Tips

Though using the essential oils mentioned in this chapter may help to support your weight loss efforts, losing weight requires the combination of many different factors. Below you will find a detailed list of general weight loss tips to help support you in your weight loss efforts.

- Pay attention to how much you are eating – most people eat much more than the recommended serving size for food which leads to a calorie excess

- Avoid snacking too much between meals – if you must snack, try something low in calories like an apple or some sliced veggies

- Make an effort to incorporate light exercise in your routine every day and moderate to intense exercise at least three times a week

- Try to reduce your intake of high-calorie, fattening foods like fast food and processed foods – this will help to reduce your daily calorie intake significantly

- Avoid using too much cooking oil when you prepare food at home as this can significantly add to the calorie content of your meal

- Do not avoid all fats – monosaturated fats like those from avocado and olive oil are very good for you

- Try to eat small meals every few hours throughout the day rather than only eating two or three large meals

- Be consistent in your exercise routine – the more often you do something the sooner it will become a habit

Essential Oil Weight Loss Wrap Recipe

Perhaps you have heard of weight loss wraps that can help to flush toxins from your body and help you to lose inches. If you go to a specialty spa, you could pay $30 or more for a single wrap. Using this recipe, not only can you save a lot of money but you can also make and use them right in your own home.

Ingredients:

1 ½ teaspoons Grapefruit essential oil

30 drops Cinnamon essential oil

30 drops Peppermint essential oil

30 drops Ginger essential oil

30 drops Lemon essential oil

Instructions:

1. Whisk together the ingredients in a small bowl and set aside.
2. Take a hot shower to open your pores and don't put any lotion on after you shower.
3. Take your measurements around your waist at the belly button as well as 2 inches above and 2 inches below.
4. Massage some of the essential oil mixture into your stomach, using strokes that move up toward your heart.
5. Wrap your stomach in a layer of light fabric like muslin then wrap with several layers of plastic wrap.
6. Leave the wrap in place for at least 45 minutes up to 8 hours.
7. Drink at least 2 glasses of water while wearing the wrap and 8 glasses the next day to help flush toxins.
8. Remove the wrap and retake your measurements.

Essential Oil Weight Loss Smoothie Recipe

Just because you want to lose weight doesn't mean you have to start a crash diet – you can make simple changes to your dietary habits and add essential oils to receive some additional benefits. This smoothie is just one of many ways you can reduce your calorie intake while boosting your nutrition and incorporating the benefits of essential oils. Enjoy this smoothie in place of lunch or breakfast to kick-start your weight loss efforts.

Ingredients:

2 cups fresh baby spinach

1 cup organic apple juice

½ cup frozen berries (your choice)

2 tablespoons chia seeds

2 tablespoons fresh lemon juice

1 teaspoon fresh grated ginger

2 drops Lemon essential oil

2 drops Grapefruit essential oil

Instructions:

1. Combine the spinach and apple juice in a blender and blend on high speed until smooth.
2. Add the remaining ingredients and blend on high speed for 30 to 60 seconds.
3. Blend in a few ice cubes, if desired, to thicken the smoothie.
4. Pour into glasses and enjoy immediately for the best benefits.

Chapter Four: Essential Oils for Beauty

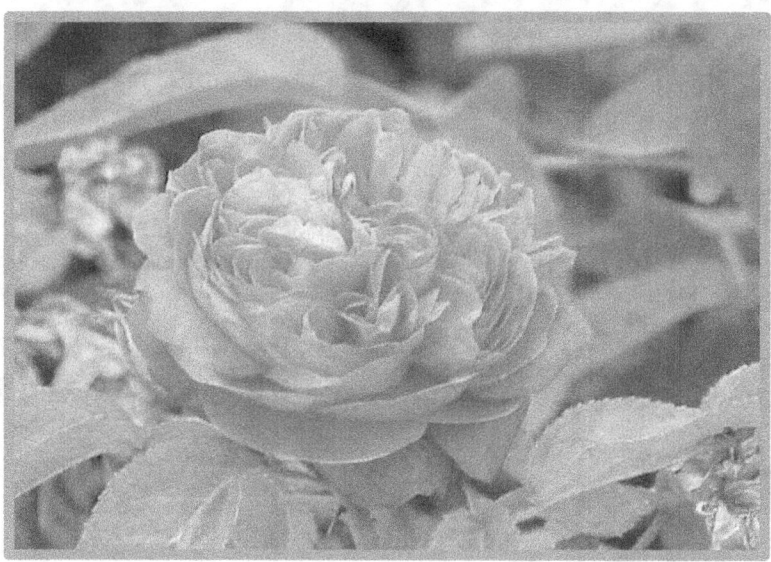

When it comes to healthy hair and skin, essential oils are loaded with natural benefits. If you pay a visit to your local health food store and check out the supply of natural beauty products, you are likely to see a lot of them made with essential oils like lavender, rose and sage. Essential oils can be used for everything from softening skin and moisturizing hair to smoothing away tension lines in your face and adding volume to your hairdo. In this chapter you will learn about some of the best essential oils for beauty and how to use them.

Some of the oils that are most beneficial for beauty include:

- Clary Sage
- Lavender
- Rose
- Geranium
- Bergamot

Clary Sage

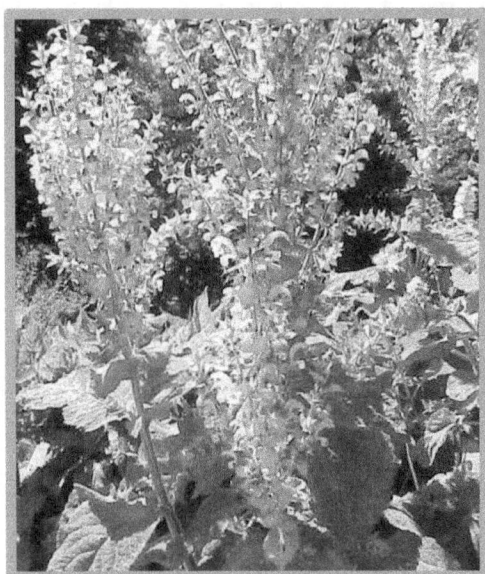 This essential oil comes from the Salvia sclarea plant and its oil is naturally high in phytoestrogens. Clary sage essential oil is typically extracted by steam distillation using the tender leaves and buds of the Clary Sage plant.

The plant is thought to be native to Europe and it has been used throughout history as a medicinal herb, known improve vision and reduce the effects of aging.

How to Use: Clary Sage essential oil can be applied topically or ingested as a dietary supplement. To use Clary Sage oil as a supplement, simply dilute one drop of oil in 4 ounces of liquid. To use this oil topically, simply apply a few drops directly to the skin and rub it in well. You can also dilute it in a carrier oil like almond oil to enhance absorption.

Components: Sclareol, Geraniol, Linalyl Acetate, Alpha Terpineol, Linalool, Neryl Acetate, Germacrene-D and Caryophyllene

Other Uses: You may be surprised to hear that Clary Sage oil can also help to ease menstrual pain and it can be very helpful for women going through menopause. Clary Sage oil has been shown to stimulate the opening of obstructed menses, easing pain and making periods more regular. This oil may also be effective in reducing irritation that often occurs when menstruation.

Blend With: blends well with citrus oils like lemon or citrus as well as lavender, sandalwood, jasmine, juniper and frankincense

<u>Lavender</u>

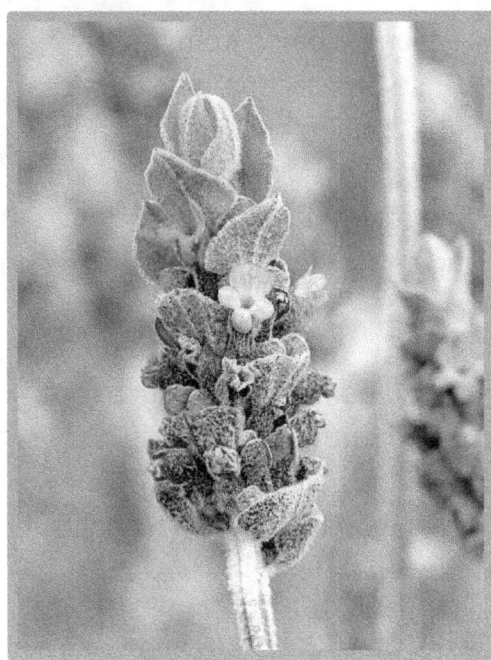

Lavender essential oil comes from the lavender plant (Lavandula) which belongs to the same family as mint. The oil of this plant has a sweet, floral scent that is very popular for aromatherapy. Lavender helps to relieve stress and tension – it may also help to balance the body.

Lavender oil is typically extracted through the process of steam distillation. In addition to its therapeutic and medicinal benefits, this oil is also very useful in making perfumes and it can be used to flavor food as well.

How to Use: Lavender essential oil is a wonderful product to use on your skin – it can also be used to heal cuts and bruises as well as skin irritation. To use this oil, rub a few drops of it directly into the skin to moisturize the area. When rubbed directly onto the skin, lavender essential oil may help reduce the appearance of scar tissue.

Components: Linalool, Linalyl Acetate, Limonene, Camphor, Caryophyllene, Lavendulyl Acetate, 3-Octanone

Other Uses: Because lavender oil is so pungent, it is often used in bug repellants – it is particularly effective against midges, mosquitos and moths. When used medicinally, lavender can also help to promote healthy sleep. It is often recommended as an alternative to sleep medication for the treatment of insomnia in elderly individuals.

Blend With: blends well with pine, clary sage, cedarwood, nutmeg and geranium

Rose

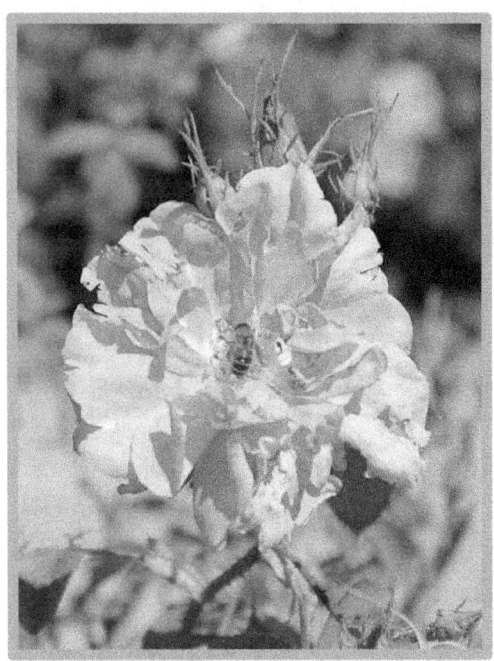

Rose essential oil typically comes from the Damascus Rose (Rosa damascene) and it has a sweet, floral scent that can be intoxicating. In addition to its usefulness in moisturizing dry skin, rose essential oil can also help to promote harmony and balance.

Though other roses can be used to produce rose essential oil, red roses like the Damascus Rose are preferred because they are particularly fragrant and red roses tend to have the highest oil content of all color varieties.

How to Use: Rose oil is especially effective as an astringent, used to strengthen the roots of your hair and to lift and tone skin. When used regularly, rose essential oil can help to prevent wrinkles and hair loss. Simply rub a few drops directly into the skin or take one drop as a supplement diluted in 4 ounces of liquid.

Components: Citonellol, Citral, Carvone, Eugenol, Ethanol, Farnesol, Stearpoten, Nerol, Nonanol, Phenyl Acetaldehyde, Phenyl Geraniol and Stearpoten

Other Uses: In addition to its uses in enhancing skin and hair health, rose essential oil can also help to balance your hormones and restore harmony in your body. The aroma of this oil has also been shown to enhance move and to improve feelings of positivity.

Blend With: blends well with jasmine, cloves, palma rosa and geranium

Geranium

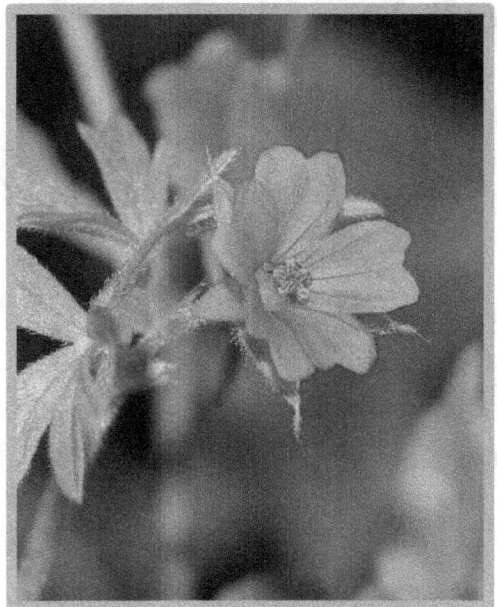

The geranium is a flowering plant that grows throughout the temperate region of the world. The flowers of this plant can be used to extract an essential oil that helps to smooth and tone skin – it is also popular in aromatherapy.

Geranium essential oil has a flowery scent that can be very uplifting – when used in aromatherapy, this oil can help to improve mood and to stimulate the release of negative memories.

How to Use: Geranium essential oil has been shown effective in treating a number of skin problems including acne, dermatitis and eczema. To use this oil, apply 2 to 4 drops to the desired area and rub it in well – unless your skin is very sensitive, you do not need to dilute the oil with a carrier oil.

Components: Alpha Pinene, Myrcene, Limonene, Menthone, Linalool, Geranyl Acetate, Citronellol, Geraniol and Geranyl Butyrate

Other Uses: In addition to its skin benefits, geranium essential oil is also known for relieving stress and depression. This oil has powerful benefits for uplifting the spirits and to improve mental function which is useful in treating depression, anxiety and anger problems. Geranium essential oil may also lessen the effects of PMS.

Blend With: blends well with angelica, bergamot, cedar, citronella, lavender, lime, orange, lemon, jasmine, grapefruit and rosemary oils

Bergamot

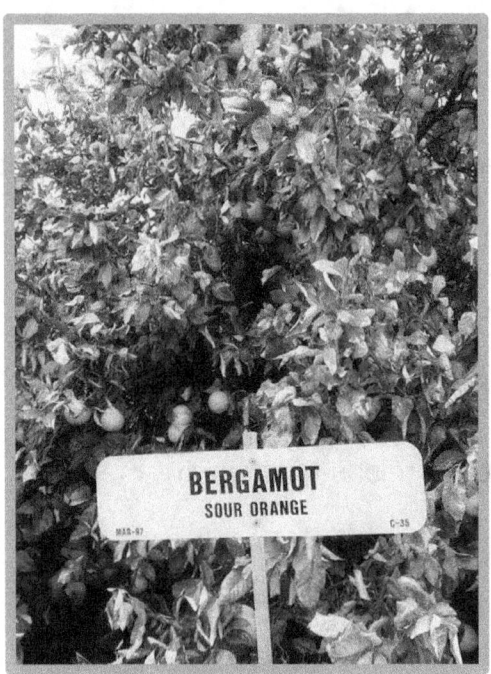

Bergamot essential oil comes from the Bergamot orange (Citrus bergamia) which is the size of a regular orange but yellow in color, like a lemon. These oranges are typically grown in Italy and the oil is usually extracted through cold-pressing.

Bergamot has a number of uses for your skin – it can help to prevent or treat cold sores, to reduce oil and to treat acne. Bergamot is also commonly used in black tea.

How to Use: Bergamot oil can be used to treat acne and to reduce the appearance of scar tissue on skin. Simply rub a drop or two directly into the skin.

Components: Alpha Pinene, Alpha Bergaptnen, Alpha Terpineol, Linalool, Limonene, Nerol, Neryl Acetate, Linalyl Acetate, Beta Bisabolene, Geraniol and Myrcene

Other Uses: In addition to its beauty benefits, Bergamot essential oil is also known for its analgesic and antibiotic properties. This oil can be used to treat pain because it stimulates the production of hormones which reduce the sensitivity of your nerves to pain. It is particularly useful in treating headaches and muscle aches.

Blend With: blends well with mandarin, jasmine, black pepper, geranium, clary sage, frankincense, rosemary and orange

Essential Oil Face Wash Recipe

Don't spend $10 or more on an expensive all-natural face wash when you can make your own right at home! Using a few simple ingredients like chamomile tea and essential oils you can make a face wash that will clear your skin without the use of any chemicals or unnatural ingredients.

Ingredients:

¼ cup liquid castile soap (organic, if possible)

¼ cup brewed chamomile tea (organic, if possible)

¾ teaspoon avocado oil

3 drops Bergamot essential oil

3 drops Rose essential oil

3 drops Lavender essential oil

Instructions:

1. Brew the chamomile tea and set ¼ cup of it aside to cool.
2. Stir together all of the ingredients in a small bowl to combine and pour into a small pump bottle
3. Use ½ to 1 teaspoon of face wash each time you wash your face and rinse with warm water.

Variations: Feel free to use different essential oils or differing amounts of those listed above according to your preference. Use any of the essential oils discussed in this chapter so you get as many skin-clearing benefits as possible.

Essential Oil Sugar Scrub Recipe

If your face is especially oily, or if you struggle with acne, you may prefer to use a facial scrub rather than a traditional face wash. This recipe is easy to throw together and will keep your face clean and clear.

Ingredients:

1 cup white sugar

½ cup almond oil

½ teaspoon Vitamin E oil

½ teaspoon pure vanilla extract

10 drops Lavender essential oil

5 drops Rose essential oil

Instructions:

1. Whisk together all of the ingredients in a mixing bowl until well combined.
2. Transfer the mixture to a small pump bottle and seal with the lid.
3. Use 1 teaspoon or so of the scrub each time you wash your face.

Variation: If you prefer a citrus scent, replace the lavender and rose essential oils with lemon and orange – use any combination of these oils up to 20 drops total.

Essential Oil Itchy Skin Relief Recipe

Whether you have a bug bite, sunburn or simply itchy skin, this recipe is definitely one you want to keep on hand. Use this spray to treat all kinds of skin irritations rather than turning to a commercial product loaded with chemicals.

Ingredients:

2 ounces Witch Hazel

5 drops Lavender essential oil

3 drops Tea Tree oil

2 drops Frankincense essential oil

Instructions:

1. Fill a 2-ounce spray bottle with Witch Hazel.
2. Add the essential oils and shake well.
3. Spritz the liquid onto your skin and gently rub it in for the maximum benefit.

Chapter Five: Essential Oils for Health

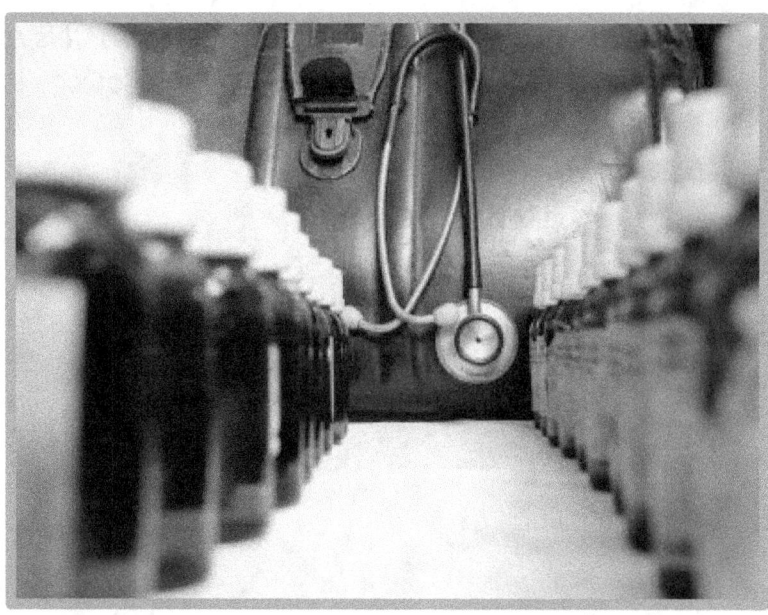

Before the development of modern medical techniques and prescription drugs, herbs and other natural substances including essential oils were used to treat minor ailments. Because you couldn't go to the grocery store to pick up a tube of Neosporin for a burn on your finger, you might rub a drop of lavender oil into the burn to soothe the skin and promote healing. If you were feeling anxious, you might drink a drop of jasmine oil diluted in tea to calm your nerves rather than getting a prescription for anti-anxiety medication. Essential oils are all-natural and they are a great way to treat minor injuries and ailments including those listed below.

Conditions that can be treated with essential oils:

- Minor cuts and scrapes
- First-degree burns (including sunburn)
- Insect bites
- Poison ivy and other skin irritation
- Upset stomach/indigestion
- Anxiety and depression
- Lack of energy

- Pain or physical discomfort
- Muscle cramps and spasms
- Menstrual pain and discomfort
- Irritability and mood swings
- Insomnia

These are just a few of the many ailments that have been treated using essential oils for thousands of years. In fact, many ancient cultures relied almost entirely on folk medicine for the treatment of common illnesses – herbs, flowers and oils were the only medicine needed. In the following pages you will learn which essential oils to use for common ailments including those listed above.

Recommended Essential Oils for Common Ailments

Over the next few pages you will discover just how versatile and amazing essential oils are. As you will see, they can be used to treat everything from depression to insomnia and everything in between.

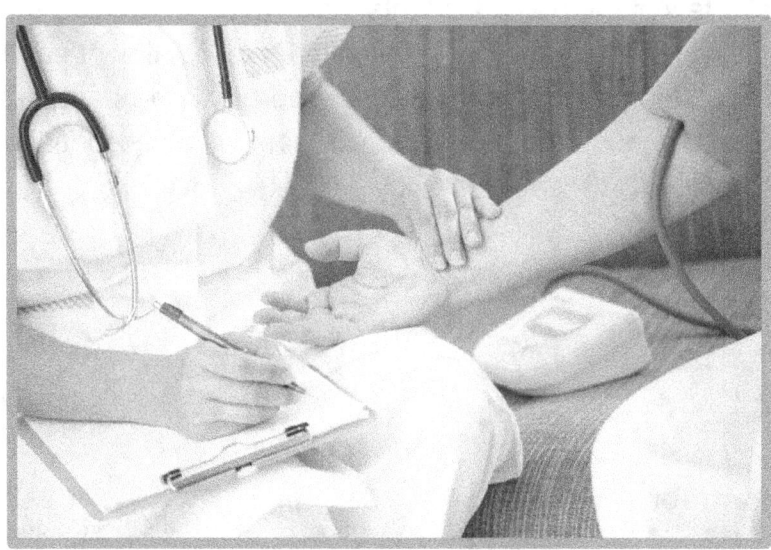

Minor Cuts and Scrapes

Small cuts and scrapes are a part of everyday life – in most cases you might just put a band-aid on it and forget about it. If you do not properly treat the wound, however, it could become infected. These essential oils help to kill germs and speed healing.

Recommended Oils: lavender, peppermint, eucalyptus, tea tree, chamomile, lemon, lime, peppermint

Minor Burns

When you get a burn, your first instinct may be to apply Neosporin or another burn cream. While these creams may provide some relief, they are not natural and may cause further irritation to your skin. Try these essential oils instead.

Recommended Oils: lavender, rose, chamomile, melrose

Cardiac Health

Many people suffer from heart conditions ranging from simple things like high blood pressure to complicated issues like heart disease and high cholesterol. These essential oils are known for providing cardiac benefits.

Recommended Oils: lemon, rosemary, wintergreen, peppermint, Cyprus, marjoram, ylang ylang, cypress

Pain Relief

Many essential oils have natural analgesic qualities – this simply means that they provide pain relief. Whether you are suffering from a headache or sore muscles, these essential oils may help.

Recommended Oils: peppermint, wintergreen, spruce, clove, tansy, nutmeg, chamomile, black pepper, rosemary, marjoram, ginger

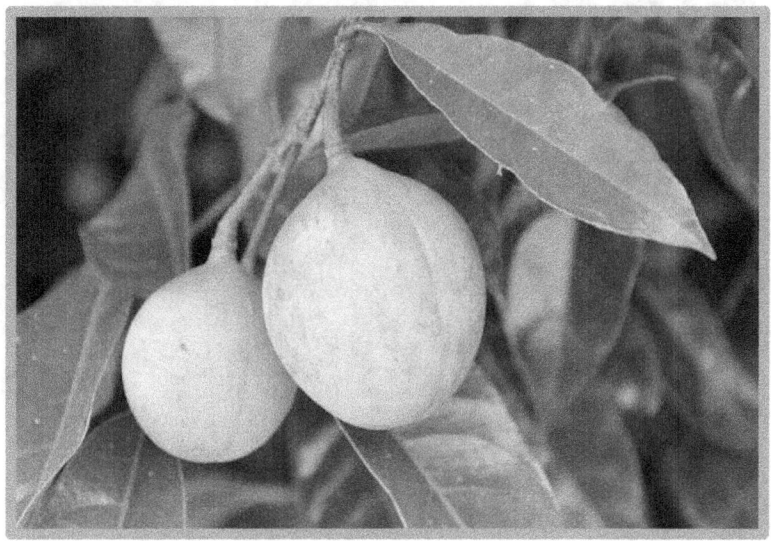

3: Nutmeg

Respiratory Health

Many people suffer from respiratory conditions ranging from simple things like a common cold to chronic issues like asthma. These essential oils are known for providing respiratory benefits.

Recommended Oils: eucalyptus, lemon, tea tree, peppermint, clary sage, oregano

Digestive Support

Whether you suffer from occasional digestive upset or you have a chronic digestive condition, these essential oils may provide some relief.

Recommended Oils: peppermint, fennel, ginger, caraway, lemongrass, clary sage, marjoram, nutmeg, clove, cardamom

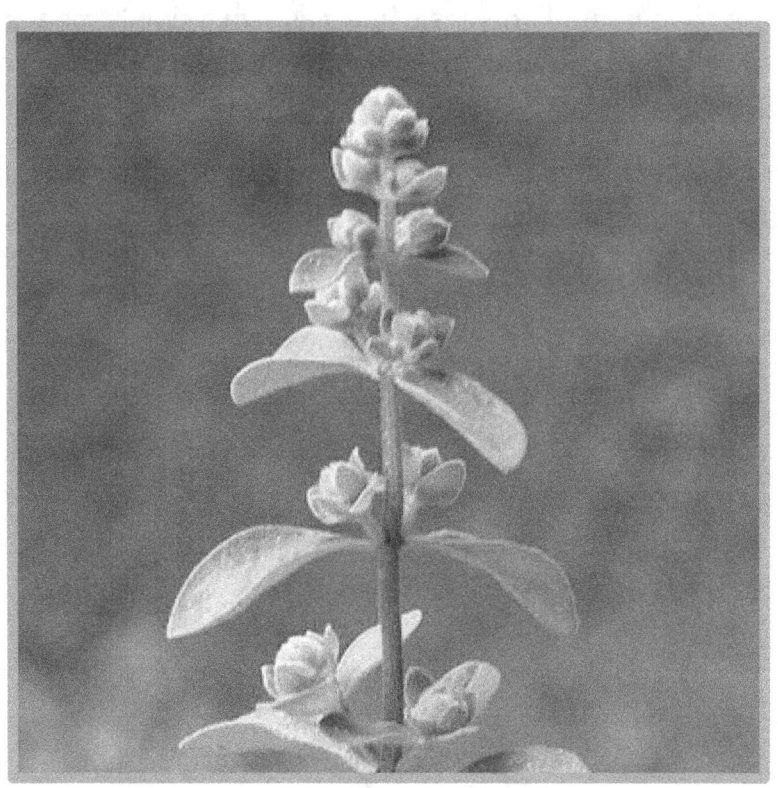

4:Marjoram

Convulsions and Spasms

Spams and convulsions can take many forms, from an epileptic seizure to an occasional muscle spasm. If you are affected by any convulsions or spasms, try these essential oils.

Recommended Oils: basil, marjoram, chamomile, clary sage, cypress, lavender, peppermint

Inflammation

There are many things that can cause inflammation including physical injuries, infections, and even the food you eat. If you are suffering from inflammation you may not need to take any medication for it – try rubbing one of these essential oils into the affected area.

Recommended Oils: thyme, cinnamon, clove, eucalyptus, fennel, bergamot, rose, peppermint, oregano, lemongrass, nutmeg

Essential Oil Burn Ointment Recipe

Whether you are suffering from a minor burn on your hand or sunburn on your entire body, this ointment is something you definitely want to keep on hand. Made with soothing essential oils and no harsh chemicals, this ointment will have you feeling better in no time.

Ingredients:

¼ cup raw honey

¼ teaspoon Lavender essential oil

2 drops Rose essential oil

Instructions:

1. Whisk together the ingredients in a small bowl.
2. Spread the ointment over the affected area in a thin layer.
3. Cover the wound with gauze.

Variation: If you are only treating a small burn, you can cut the recipe in half – use only 2 tablespoons of honey and 1/8 teaspoon Lavender essential oil with one drop of rose essential oil.

Essential Oils for Mental Health

Sometimes we get so caught up in treating the physical symptoms of illness that we forget to take care of our mind and spirit. Essential oils have a number of extraordinary benefits for both the body and mind, so don't overlook them if you suffer from common mental issues including fatigue, depression and anxiety. Below you will find a list of essential oils that can be beneficial in treating a variety of mental and emotional problems.

Stress and Anxiety

Whether you are having a particularly stressful week at work or you suffer from an anxiety disorder, these essential oils will help to ease your mind and calm your anxiety in a natural way.

Recommended Oils: chamomile, geranium, lavender, marjoram, sandalwood, bergamot, orange, tangerine, rosemary and thyme

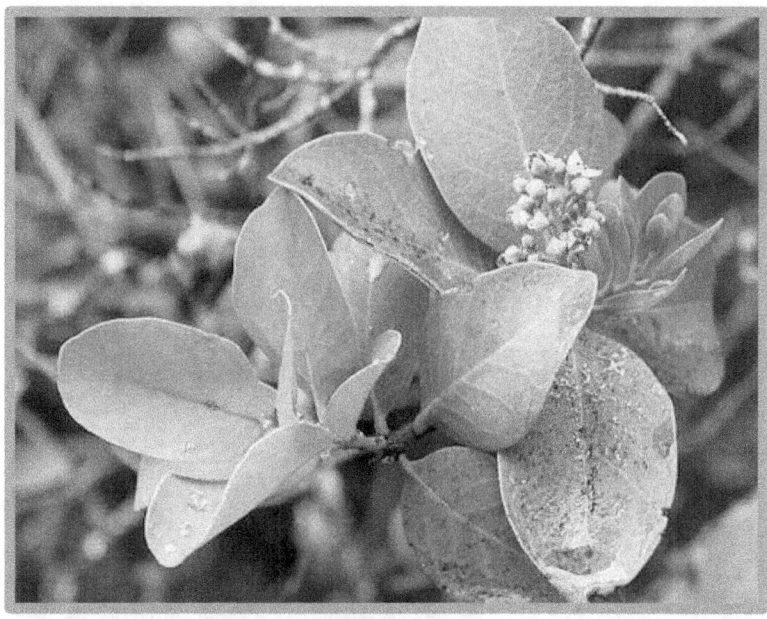

5: Sandalwood

Depression

Many people suffer from depression but there is such a large stigma against mental illness that most do not seek treatment. If you suffer from mild or occasional depression, these essential oils may help.

Recommended Oils: jasmine, sandalwood, clary sage, bergamot, rose, geranium, ylang ylang, petitgrain

Insomnia

If you have trouble sleeping, you may find that it affects you both physically and mentally. Taking over-the-counter sleep aids or even prescription drugs may do more harm than good, so give these essential oils a try instead.

Recommended Oils: lavender, chamomile, sandalwood, marjoram

Mood Disorders

Many people suffer from occasional irritability or mood swings, but you don't have to suffer any longer. These essential oils may help to balance out your mood, helping you to feel more positive.

Recommended Oils: lemon, jasmine, lavender, rosemary, cinnamon, peppermint

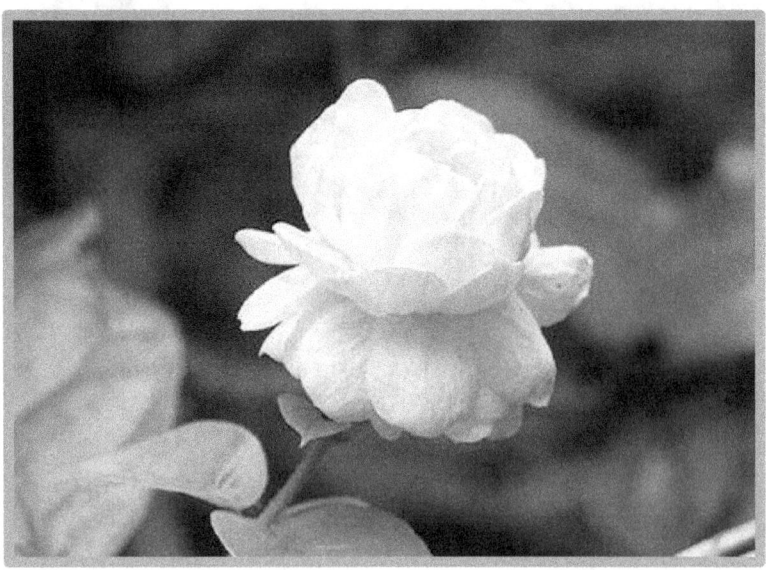

6: Jasmine

Inner Peace

If you feel as though your mind is constantly out of balance or you are looking for a way to enhance your meditation, try some of these essential oils.

Recommended Oils: orange, rose, clove, lavender, geranium, patchouli, mandarin, sage, sandalwood, frankincense

Lack of Focus

If you have a hard time focusing on work, school, or other things, you do not necessarily have to down energy drinks or seek a prescription. These essential oils have been shown to help improve cognitive function and focus.

Recommended Oils: rosemary, basil, juniper, peppermint, clary sage

Chapter Six: Other Uses for Essential Oil

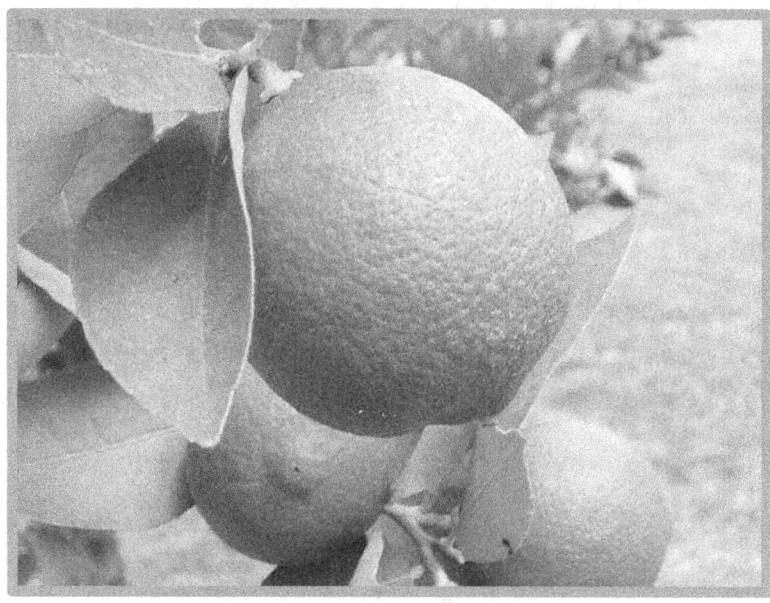

As you may know by now, essential oils are very versatile – they can be used for a variety of purposes. While many essential oils are used for aromatherapy or as natural remedies for minor ailments, these are not the only things they are good for. Some essential oils, for example, can be used to make your own cleaning products and bug repellants. Below you will find a list of alternative uses for essential oils and, in the following pages, instructions for these methods.

Other uses for essential oils include:

- Homemade bug spray to repel mosquitos
- All-natural cleaning products
- Chemical-free pesticides for plants
- Easy odor control for the home

Cleaning Products from Essential Oils

When it comes to keeping your home clean, you need a product that works well and will keep your family safe. Unfortunately, many commercial cleaning products are laced with toxic ingredients like chemicals that can be harmful to your children and pets. If you want to avoid these chemicals, try making your own cleaning products at home. Below you will find recipes for several basic cleaning products including a kitchen sink scrub, an all-purpose disinfectant and an odor-repellant.

Kitchen Sink Scrub

Use this scrub to clean the water stains and food residue from your kitchen sink – it will leave it sparkling clean.

Ingredients:

½ cup baking soda

2 tablespoons distilled white vinegar

5 drops Bergamot essential oil

5 drops Lime essential oil

Instructions:

1. Combine all of the ingredients in a small bowl and stir until well combined in a thick paste.
2. Use the paste to scrub your kitchen sink then wash with warm water.

<u>All-Purpose Disinfectant Cleaner</u>

This disinfectant is mild enough to use on kitchen counters but strong enough to kill even the nastiest of germs.

Ingredients:

1 clean dish cloth

Hot water

3 drops Lemon essential oil

Instructions:

1. Place a dish cloth in a bowl of hot water and add a few drops of Lemon essential oil.
2. Let the cloth soak overnight then use it to clean and disinfect common surfaces.

<u>Odor-Repellant</u>

This odor repellant is so easy that you can use it anywhere in your house – use it to deodorize a smelly trash can or use it in your garage to clear out nasty odors.

Ingredients:

Cotton balls

Peppermint, spearmint or pine essential oil

Instructions:

1. Place a few drops of essential oil on cotton balls and place them where needed.

Homemade Bug Spray Recipe

Commercial bug sprays are loaded with chemicals and other nasty ingredients that can leave your skin dry and itchy. This recipe is an excellent alternative for all-natural and homemade bug spray that works incredibly well. Make sure you keep this recipe on hand throughout the summer!

Ingredients:

4 ounces boiling water

3 ½ ounces Witch Hazel

½ teaspoon vegetable glycerin

10 drops Lemongrass essential oil

10 drops Rosemary essential oil

10 drops Eucalyptus essential oil

10 drops Lavender essential oil

Instructions:

1. Place the boiling water and Witch Hazel in an 8-ounce spray bottle.
2. Add the vegetable glycerin as well as the essential oils and shake well.
3. Spritz the liquid over your skin to repel insects.

Substitutions: You can use any combination of essential oils for this recipe – you only need a total of 30 to 50 drops. Some of the oils you might use include eucalyptus, lemongrass, citronella, clove, rosemary, tea tree, cedar, catnip, lavender and mint

All-Natural Pesticide for Plants

If you find that your garden is riddled with insect pests, don't run to the garden supply store and buy a commercial pesticide. These pesticides contain harmful chemicals that can contaminate the vegetables and herbs you put on your family's table. Using all-natural essential oils you can make your own homemade pesticide for plants.

Ingredients:

8 ounces distilled water

1 ½ tablespoons liquid dish soap

3 drops Spearmint essential oil

3 drops Citronella essential oil

3 drops Lavender essential oil

3 drops Cedar essential oil

Instructions:

Combine the water and dish soap in an 8-ounce spray bottle.

Add the essential oils and shake gently.

Spray the liquid on your plants and vegetables to repel insect pests.

Optional Additions: To protect your plants from mildew and fungus, add 4 drops of lemon or orange essential oil to the mixture.

Conclusion

Hopefully after reading this book you have a clear understanding of what essential oils are and what they can do. Not only can essential oils be used as cleaning products or in aromatherapy, but they also have medicinal a therapeutic benefits. In reading this book you have received some valuable tips on how to use some of the most popular essential oils including lemon, lavender, eucalyptus and rose. Give some of these oils a try and see the benefits for yourself!

Also check out my other title below

Canning and Preserving at Home - Delicious Sauces, Jellies, Relishes, Chutneys, Salsas, Pie fillings and more!

http://www.amazon.com/dp/B00KBIL5CS

Thanks for reading and have fun using essential oils to meet your goals!

Like this book? Please leave a review.

References

"21 Things You Should Know About Essential Oils." Crunchy Betty.
<http://www.crunchybetty.com/21-things-you-should-know-about-essential-oils>

"About Essential Oils." Young Living.
<http://www.youngliving.com/en_US/discover/guide/about>

Crane, Stephanie. "Lose Inches with DIY Body Wraps." Stephanie Blue.
<http://stephanieblue.com/slim-sassy-body-wrap/>

"Do It Yourself: All-Natural Garden Pesticide Spray." Young Living Blog.
<https://blog.youngliving.com/do-it-yourself-all-natural-garden-pesticide-spray/#.U4jxofldWh0>

"Essential Oils: Hazards, Warnings and Guidelines." Mountain Rose Herbs.
<https://www.mountainroseherbs.com/learn/essential-oils-warning>

Hupston, Fleur. "Heal with Traditional Home and Folk Remedies of Nature." Natural News. <http://www.naturalnews.com/028501_folk_remedies_self_healing.html>

Kynes, Sandra. "The History of Herbal Medicine and Essential Oils." UTNE Reader.
<http://www.utne.com/mind-and-body/history-of-herbal-medicine-ze0z1404zcov.aspx#axzz33DNf5gD9>

Photo Credits

Alembic, Photo by David Darling,
<http://www.daviddarling.info/encyclopedia/A/alembic.html>

Bergamot Orange, Photo by Leslie Seaton via Wikimedia Commons,
<http://en.wikipedia.org/wiki/File:Bergamot_-_Sour_Orange_(Tree)_-_Waddell,_Maricopa_County,_Arizona,_USA_-_January_2013.jpg>

Bulgarian Rose, Photo by Edal Anton Lefterov via Wikimedia Commons,
<http://en.wikipedia.org/wiki/File:Bulgarian_Rosa_damascena.JPG>

Cedar Shoot, Photo by MPF via Wikimedia Commons,
<http://en.wikipedia.org/wiki/File:Cedrus_libani_shoot.jpg>

Chamomile, Photo by Kallerna via Wikimedia Commons,
<http://en.wikipedia.org/wiki/File:Kamomillasaunio_(Matricaria_recutita).JPG>

Cinnamon, Photo by Thiry via Wikimedia Commons,
<http://en.wikipedia.org/wiki/File:Baton_de_cannelle.jpg>

Citrus Blossom, Photo by Ellen Levy Finch via Wikimedia Commons,
<http://en.wikipedia.org/wiki/File:OrangeBloss_wb.jpg>

Clary Sage, Photo by Chris73 via Wikimedia Commons,
<http://en.wikipedia.org/wiki/File:Salvia_sclarea3.jpg>

Damascus Rose, Photo by Sony Mavica via Wikimedia Commons,
<http://en.wikipedia.org/wiki/File:Rosa_damascena5.jpg>

Eucalyptus, Photo by Ethel Aardvark via Wikimedia Commons, <http://en.wikipedia.org/wiki/File:Eucalyptus_tereticornis_flowers,_capsules,_buds_and_foliage.jpeg>

Geranium, Photo by Alvesgaspar via Wikimedia Commons, <http://en.wikipedia.org/wiki/File:Geranium_February_2008-1.jpg>

Ginger, Photo by Venkatx5 via Wikimedia Commons, <http://en.wikipedia.org/wiki/File:Ginger_Plant_vs.jpg>

Grapefruit, Photo by Lipsio via Wikimedia Commons, <http://en.wikipedia.org/wiki/File:Grapefruit.ebola.jpeg>

Jasmine, Photo by Scott Zona via Wikimedia Commons, <http://en.wikipedia.org/wiki/File:Jasminum_sambac_%27Grand_Duke_of_Tuscany%27.jpg>

Lavender, Photo by Riley Huntley via Wikimedia Commons, <http://commons.wikimedia.org/wiki/File:Lavender_7.JPG>

Lavender Flower, Photo by Fir0002 via Wikimedia Commons, <http://en.wikipedia.org/wiki/File:Single_lavendar_flower02.jpg>

Lemon, Photo by Elena Chochkova via Wikimedia Commons, <http://en.wikipedia.org/wiki/File:P1030323.JPG>

Lime, Photo by Wtstoffs via Wikimedia Commons, <http://en.wikipedia.org/wiki/File:Backyard_limes.jpg>

Marjoram, Photo by Dobromila via Wikimedia Commons,
<http://en.wikipedia.org/wiki/File:Majeranek2.jpg>

Nutmeg, Photo by Joe Ravi via Wikimedia Commons,
<http://en.wikipedia.org/wiki/File:Nutmeg_on_Tree.jpg>

Peppermint, Photo by Sten Porse via Wikimedia Commons,
<http://en.wikipedia.org/wiki/File:Mentha-piperita.JPG>

Rose Water, Photo by Marc Smith via Wikimedia Commons,
<http://en.wikipedia.org/wiki/File:Rose_petals_afloat.jpg>

Sandalwood, Photo by KarlM via Wikimedia Commons,
<http://en.wikipedia.org/wiki/File:Santalum_paniculatum_1326.jpg>

www.ingramcontent.com/pod-product-compliance
Lightning Source LLC
Chambersburg PA
CBHW081754280526
45789CB00008B/2857